SYNOPS.. THE MENOPAUSE MANIFESTO

Own your health with facts and feminism by Jen Gunter

Dr. Camilla Gary

TABLE OF CONTENT

TABLE OF CONTENT

INTRODUCTION

SYNOPSIS ONE

UNDERERSTANDING YOUR BODY AS A WOMAN

SYNOPSIS TWO

WHAT TO ENCOUNTER WHEN EXPECTING MENOPAUSE
WHAT IS MENOPAUSE?

SYNOPSIS THREE

WHAT ARE SOME INTEGRATIVE TREATMENTS AND RECUPERATING PRACTICES TO CONSIDER FOR MENOPAUSE?
INSTRUCTIONS TO UTILIZE INTEGRATIVE TREATMENTS IN MENOPAUSE AND PERIMENOPAUSE

SYNOPSIS FOUR

TAKING CHARGE OF THE CHANGE IN YOU

CONCLUTION

INTRODUCTION

Menopause is something each lady will insight into, yet it is a theme so infrequently spoken about. As a lady, you ought to consistently realize what's in store with regards to your own body–particularly as it ages. This is the reason we've composed *synopsis of The Menopause Manifesto*: all you require to think about menopause, its regular indications, menopause treatment, and the various periods of menopause.

Very many like little youngsters go through adolescence, ladies go through another significant progress with their bodies in middle age called menopause. Estrogen and progesterone creation from female regenerative organs begin to ease off, and periods in the long run stop.

As ladies age, their chemical levels normally start to diminish and their ovaries quit delivering eggs–in this way, they quit having periods and cannot, at this point become pregnant. Most of the ladies go through menopause in their 40s and 50s, although everybody's body is unique.

To place it in clinical terms, menopause is essential for a characteristic natural cycle in which period and fruitfulness stop for ladies. Menopause shows itself through actual results, however, it can likewise massively affect emotional well-being and in general prosperity. In *synopsis of The Menopause Manifesto*, you'll figure out how to expect the signs and manifestations of menopause and successfully treat them.

SYNOPSIS ONE

UNDERERSTANDING YOUR BODY AS A WOMAN

Sound sexual and regenerative organs are essential to a lady's sexual wellbeing. Finding out about the elements of every organ and how these organs cooperate permits you to know about your body and any progressions that may show an issue. This data can likewise assist you with picking a strategy for conception prevention or decide when the best and ideal opportunity to attempt to get pregnant is.

Finding out about a lady's sexual reactions may likewise make you more alright with your body. If you comprehend what befalls your body when you are physically energized, you might have the option to improve your sexual encounters.

A lady's sexual reactions change for the duration of her life cycle. To some extent, this is because of her changing degrees of involvement and self-information, yet there are additionally actual changes as her body develops. Pregnancy and labor may affect a lady's sexual reactions. Managing the physical and passionate changes related to menopause is likewise a significant piece of a lady's sexual wellbeing.

THE INTERIOR ORGANS

The biggest organ in the female regenerative framework is the uterus. More often than not it is moderately little, about the size of your clench hand. In a typical pregnancy, the embryo creates inside the uterus, extending it to commonly its ordinary size. Visit the pregnancy virtual wellbeing community to study this subject.

On the two sides of the uterus are pockets called ovaries. The ovaries contain unfertilized eggs or ova. At the point when one of these ova (called an ovum) joins with a man's sperm, it is prepared and may ultimately deliver a youngster.

A young lady's ovaries start delivering ova at adolescence provoking the beginning of her periods.

At the point when the ovaries quit creating ova, a lady has arrived at menopause. Cylinders connected to the ovaries are called Fallopian tubes permitting the ovum to venture out to the uterus.

The vagina interfaces the uterus to the outside of the body. This entry has a few significant capacities for ladies:

a man's penis may enter a lady's vagina during sex (Vaginal entrance by a penis is called intercourse. Intercourse is the most likely path for a lady to get pregnant. Fingers or other clean articles may likewise enter the vagina during sexual play. Every lady is special in her happiness regarding sex. Choosing what gives us joy is a significant piece of finding out about our sexual selves).

feminine blood is helped out of the body through the vagina

at the point when a child is conveyed typically, it goes through the vagina

At the point when the vagina of a grown-up lady is solid, it contains numerous sorts of innocuous microorganisms. A portion of these microbes are like those found on the skin, yet different microscopic organisms called lactobacilli are discovered principally in the vagina. These microbes help shield the vagina from diseases with yeast and different microorganisms.

The association between the uterus and the vagina is known as the cervix. This is a tight opening, which shields the uterus from outside pollutants.

THE OUTER ORGANS

The clitoris is the conceptive organ generally associated with sexual joy. The top piece of the clitoris is a short projection over the vaginal opening. Notwithstanding, the greater part of the clitoris is inside the body. Its tip is touchy, so the clitoris is secured by a fold of skin called the hood. Blood hurries to the clitoris when a lady is physically excited, making it the main organ for a female sexual reaction.

Between the clitoris and the vagina is the little opening associated with the urethra. A lady pees from this opening.

Folds of skin called the labia secure the clitoris and the vaginal opening.

THE FEMININE CYCLE

Changes in a lady's chemicals that happen each month direct her body to deliver a minuscule egg or ovum. The various stages in the creation of this ovum are utilized to portray a lady's period. By and large, the body delivers an ovum once at regular intervals and this is the normal length of a monthly cycle. A few ladies have longer or more limited cycles.

A lady's monthly cycle starts with her period. To quantify your own feminine cycle, record the date of the primary day you see blood during your period. The time from the main draining day of one period to the principal draining day of the following time frame is the length of your feminine cycle.

Ladies as a rule start having periods in their initial adolescents, however, a lady's periods can begin as right on time as age 9 or as late as 16 or 17. Having a period implies that a lady's monthly cycles have started and that she can become pregnant if the ovum she delivers joins with a man's sperm.

CHANGES IN YOUR CYCLE

Now and again a lady's cycles are sporadic, which implies they come at an alternate time each month. This is especially regular for young people, nonetheless, most ladies miss a period or experience different varieties in their cycle eventually in their lives. You may miss a period because:

you are pregnant

your body is as yet developing

you are under pressure at work, home, or school

you are moving toward menopause

you've been practicing enthusiastically

you've lost a ton of weight in a brief timeframe

you have a chemical problem

you've been utilizing remedy or road drugs

Albeit a portion of these progressions is essential for a lady's normal life cycle it is consistently shrewd to talk about changes in your period with your primary care physician.

THE PHASES OF THE MONTHLY CYCLE

Two significant chemicals oversee the period:

estrogen

progesterone

Chemicals are synthetic couriers, which the body uses to send directions starting with one piece of the body then onto the next. The degrees of estrogen and progesterone signal the progressions that occur during the feminine cycle. Recollect that these chemicals additionally impact different pieces of the body. For instance, estrogen assists a lady in withholding calcium in her bones. The impact of these chemicals is likewise thought to cause a large number of the side effects of premenstrual conditions.

SYNOPSIS TWO

WHAT TO ENCOUNTER WHEN EXPECTING MENOPAUSE

WHAT IS MENOPAUSE?

Many characterize menopause as the interaction that happens when a lady hasn't had a period for 12 straight months (and isn't pregnant nor wiped out). Yet, menopause is significantly more than that. It's a normal piece of maturing for females. Ladies going through a medical procedure to eliminate their uterus or ovaries for certain clinical reasons (e.g., malignancy, endometriosis, and so forth) will encounter menopause.

THE PHASES OF MENOPAUSE

There are three particular phases of menopause and each accompanies its own arrangement of side effects:

PERIMENOPAUSE

Per menopause starts to happen somewhere in the range of three to five years before real menopause. It is the cycle by which chemical levels start to drop. Most of the ladies begin encountering per menopause in their late 40s. Many mistake menopause for per menopause, as this is the stage where the normal manifestations are hot blazes, sleep deprivation, raised pulse, and emotional episodes. Periods likewise become considerably more unpredictable during this stage with the feminine stream getting either lighter or heavier. Ladies can get pregnant during this stage; in any case, it is undeniably more uncertain.

MENOPAUSE

Menopause is the stage after per menopause when ladies don't bleed for an entire year. Getting to this point can take on normal somewhere in the range of one to three years, and it differs relying upon the person.

POSTMENOPAUSE

This is the stage that comes after it has been an entire year since the last period cycle.

During this period, ladies frequently keep on encountering side effects like hot glimmers, night sweats, urinary issues, raised pulse, and emotional episodes.

At what age does menopause start?

The interaction of menopause will appear to be unique for each lady. There are a few factors that decide when female beginnings encountering menopause, with the greatest one being hereditary qualities for example the age of the lady's mom when she encountered menopause.

Studies have discovered planning with menopause to be vigorously hereditarily decided. One, specifically, showed the up to 20 percent of ladies that accomplished early menopause likewise had family members that had encountered it.

Early menopause additionally happens when a lady encounters ovarian disappointment, or with medical procedures like hysterectomy (evacuation of the uterus) and oophorectomies (expulsion of the ovaries). Furthermore, malignancy medicines like chemotherapy can influence the regenerative framework and cause ladies to arrive at menopause prior.

In any case, the accompanying (as opposed to prevalent thinking) have not been found to affect the age a lady starts menopause:

• The age of the lady during her first feminine period

• Pregnancy and number of pregnancies

• Whether the lady breastfed or not

• Hormonal contraception techniques

It's imperative to monitor your monthly cycle and wellbeing side effects especially as you age. Make a point to go for customary registration where the specialist will check your blood and chemical levels for any anomalies.

How long does menopause last?

The three unique stages of menopause can last a couple of years–up to five as a rule. Once more, the interaction is diverse for every individual lady relying upon the condition of her wellbeing and hereditary cosmetics. Some may start to encounter per menopause ten years before their last period, and others may have it finished within a year–everything truly depends.

What befalls your body during menopause?

During menopause, there is a significant change occurring with the chemical levels in the body. The entirety of the actual manifestations of menopause is brought about by the change in chemical levels. It's critical to know what the basic indications are and get some information about them.

Likewise, it's imperative to take note that while your body is going through changes, menopause isn't a sickness, nor does it mean the finish of your sexuality. Here are a few changes that will happen:

- Irregular periods
- Lower levels of the accompanying chemicals:
- Estrogen
- Progesterone
- Testosterone
- Follicle-invigorating chemical (FSH)
- Luteinizing chemical (LH)
- Loss of dynamic ovarian follicles

WHAT ARE THE EARLY INDICATIONS OF MENOPAUSE?

The beginnings of menopause normally start in ladies in the late 30s when the ovaries start to make less estrogen and progesterone. Numerous ladies start to see changes in their monthly cycle in their mid-40s. It will be not quite the same as individual to individual.

Likewise remember that uncommon conditions like a hysterectomy, chemotherapy, untimely ovarian disappointment, or other ailments will welcome menopause sooner.

What are the manifestations of menopause?

Indications of menopause fluctuate from one individual to another, and every manifestation itself can have various degrees of power. It's likewise essential to recall that menopause indications don't simply appear as physical yet passionate also. Here is an overall rundown of the variety of indications any lady going through menopause may insight:

- Irregular periods
- Loss of moxie
- Mood swings
- Lack of energy
- Hot streaks
- Sweating
- Racing heart
- Headaches
- Dizziness
- Vaginal dryness
- Hair misfortune/hair diminishing
- Pain during sex

- Insomnia
- Concentration trouble
- Lapses in memory
- Weight acquire and swelling
- Breast torment/delicacy
- Digestive issues
- Depression and uneasiness
- Osteoporosis
- Dry skin
- Painful joints

A medical issue like sickness, hysterectomy, disease therapies, or smoking can intensify a portion of these menopause side effects. Additionally, every lady's menopause experience is remarkable to her. One individual may encounter an enormous scope of manifestations, while another might encounter just two. Make certain to screen your own progressions in your body and do whatever it takes not to gauge your own menopause experience against another lady. On the off chance that you feel like something uncommon is occurring, you ought to consistently talk with your primary care physician.

WHAT IS A HOT GLIMMER?

An expected 75% of ladies experience hot glimmers while going through menopause. A hot glimmer is a point at which you out of nowhere feel warm or hot, trailed by feeling cold. Commonly, the skin flushes and the heart beats quicker. Hot glimmers that happen during rest are named night sweats.

While hot glimmers shift from one lady to another, they frequently last around one to two minutes. They can be gentle or extreme and change in recurrence relying upon the lady.

A few ladies may keep on encountering hot glimmers as they go into post menopause, however, certain prescriptions can likewise welcome them on.

What sort of inconveniences are there?

A chosen handful of ladies may encounter difficulties from menopause. While our expectation isn't to frighten you, it's essential to see any unusual changes in your body and carry them to your primary care physician for assessment. That way, any complexities you experience can be managed proficiently. These can include:

- Vulvovaginal decay
- Painful intercourse
- Slowed metabolic capacity
- Cardiovascular sickness
- Osteoporosis
- Periodontal sickness
- Cataracts;
- and more

Treating menopause indications

Fortunately, there are numerous approaches to treat the indications of menopause. One of the primary significant things individuals can do is to eat an eating routine wealthy in leafy foods, calcium, and entire grain. A decent benchmark is consistently significant.

For ladies experiencing extreme manifestations, chemical treatment may be an alternative recommended by your PCP. Chemical treatment therapy can help decrease the power of hot glimmers and night sweats, vaginal decay, osteoporosis, and that's just the beginning.

Different kinds of drug that can be issues to help improve:

- Topical medicines for balding
- Lubricant for vaginal dryness
- Sleep drugs
- Antibiotics for UTIs
- Medication for osteoporosis

Some other common approaches to treat menopause incorporate reflection, needle therapy, and other unwinding procedures notwithstanding a solid eating routine joined with satisfactory exercise. For the passionate pieces of menopause, it very well may be useful to discover support through a companion, bunch, specialist, online local area, or a blend of those things.

SYNOPSIS THREE

WHAT ARE SOME INTEGRATIVE TREATMENTS AND RECUPERATING PRACTICES TO CONSIDER FOR MENOPAUSE?

From a comprehensive point of view, menopause isn't an ailment, yet a day-to-day existence change through which all ladies pass. Notwithstanding, that doesn't reject that there are unfortunate manifestations in some cases.

Integrative treatments for menopause mean to facilitate the troubles of awkward side effects. The utilization of integrative treatments for menopause manifestations is normal. Ladies who use them, for the most part, discover them to be useful. A phone review of over 850 ladies age 45 to 65 showed that 76% utilized elective treatments, including 22% who utilized them to treat their menopause side effects. Also, upwards of 89% detailed that they discovered these treatments to be "fairly" or accommodating.

While separated mediations, like a natural medication or needle therapy, may facilitate an inconvenience like hot glimmers, confined side effect treatment alone isn't the sole expectation of an integrative methodology. Incorporated methodologies center around bringing the body into ideal equilibrium, which will normally lessen the actual inconvenience. This includes mental, enthusiastic, and otherworldly equilibrium also, which is a sound objective for any period of life, including menopause.

PSYCHE/BODY PRACTICES

Clinical investigations that have analyzed the effect of activity, reformist muscle unwinding, unwinding breathing, guided relaxations, and stress the executives rehearses in menopausal and premenopausal ladies have not discovered an explicit decrease in the particular protests of hot blazes, night sweats, vaginal dryness, or rest unsettling influences. In any case, there is improvement in generally speaking personal satisfaction, which is a significant objective.

Menopause is an ideal chance to analyze one's life, to discover articulation and fulfillment with work and connections, and to feel focused on an option that could be bigger than ourselves—to discover the reason.

It is an incredible chance to develop self-intelligent practices, like reflection and journaling. There are numerous magnificent assets about this season of life, including The Second 50% of Life, by Angeles Arians, Ph.D.; and The Shrewdness of Menopause: Making Physical and Enthusiastic Wellbeing and Mending During the Change, and The Mysterious Delights of Menopause, both by Christiane Northrup, MD.

BOTANICALS AND ENHANCEMENTS

Most plant supplements utilized for menopause are thought to give benefits through dynamic fixings that go about as phytoestrogens-plant substances that behave like estrogen in the body. Nonetheless, the exploration is blended with the outcomes.

Run-of-the-mill dosages for every herbal are demonstrated beneath. Nonetheless, you should converse with your medical services supplier before adding botanicals to your wellbeing routine and get some information about the correct dose for you.

• Soy in the eating regimen has not been appeared in preliminaries to improve indications better than fake treatment.

• Is flavones (avg. 50 mg/day), in very much done examinations, have not been demonstrated to be superior to fake treatment at improving explicit menopausal manifestations, albeit some momentary investigations propose improvement in hot blazes.

• Many over-the-counter items join numerous botanicals to accomplish ideal impact, and such blends have not been very much considered.

• Red clover (40-160 mg/day) has additionally not been exceptional than fake treatment in investigations.

• Black cohosh is quite possibly the most well-known over-the-counter botanicals. Early exploration recommends 40mg/day will improve hot blazes. Notwithstanding, there are worries about liver poisonousness and conceivable effect on bosom tumor advancement in creature models.

NATUROPATHIC MEDICATION

Naturopathic medication might be a decent methodology for ladies who want a characteristic and integrative way to deal with menopause, with direction and backing for diet, way of life, botanicals, hydrotherapy, and different apparatuses.

In one deliberate investigation of Naturopathy versus customary clinical treatment for menopausal ladies, Naturopathy gave off an impression of being a powerful other option, giving tantamount help of explicit menopausal indications contrasted with ordinary treatment.

CONVENTIONAL CHINESE MEDICATION

Conventional Chinese Medication suppliers work with ladies to streamline their nourishment, action, and interior lively equilibrium, utilizing spices, needle therapy, development rehearses (Qigong and Jujitsu), rub (Tui Na), and different procedures. Momentary examinations about needle therapy alone have not shown an advantage in diminishing hot blazes, however, the entire framework's approach has not been very much assessed. A one-to two-month preliminary with a TCM supplier may give you a sign of whether this methodology is helpful for you.

HOMEOPATHY

Homeopathy is another methodology utilized by certain ladies to help oversee indications. A 2010 outline of examination on homeopathy and menopause discovered blended outcomes, with a huge level of ladies in certain investigations announcing improvement in indications, while two little clinical preliminaries discovered no measurably huge improvement. The rundown reasons that very much planned preliminaries of homeopathy for menopause side effects are required.

INSTRUCTIONS TO UTILIZE INTEGRATIVE TREATMENTS IN MENOPAUSE AND PERIMENOPAUSE

Likewise with any clinical "condition," instructing oneself is of most extreme significance. Find out about the progressions occurring in your body during menopause. Studies show that ladies who get instructive advising in menopause are less inclined to erroneously credit actual torment objections to menopause.

It is imperative to find out about the optional impacts of menopause, like osteoporosis, expanded coronary illness hazard, and cognitive decline that may potentially be forestalled through explicit medicines.

On the off chance that you utilize plant supplements, particularly on the off chance that you are likewise utilizing drugs, it is imperative to educate your medical care supplier.

Each lady has an alternate per menopause experience. Not all ladies experience hazardous side effects and the individuals who do encounter indications to various degrees. Monitor your repetitive issues, when they happen, and what elements sway them so you can roll out essential improvements.

In particular, recollect that menopause is a characteristic period of life. You may need assistance with manifestations for a period, yet you ordinarily will not need help for the remainder of your life.

Menopause and Great Sustenance

Some dangerous elements and manifestations connected with maturing and menopause can't be changed. However, great sustenance can help forestall or facilitate certain conditions that may create during and after menopause.

FUNDAMENTAL DIETARY RULES FOR MENOPAUSE

During menopause, eat an assortment of food varieties to get every one of the supplements you need. Since ladies' weight control plans are frequently low in iron and calcium, follow these rules:

Get sufficient calcium. Eat and drink two to four servings of dairy items and calcium-rich food varieties daily. Calcium is found in dairy items, fish with bones (like sardines and canned salmon), broccoli, and vegetables. Mean to get 1,200 milligrams each day.

Siphon up your iron. Eat at any rate three servings of iron-rich food sources a day. Iron is found in lean red meat, poultry, fish, eggs, verdant green vegetables, nuts, and advanced grain items. The suggested dietary recompense for iron in more established ladies is 8 milligrams per day.

Get sufficient fiber. Take food sources high in fiber, for example, entire grain bread, cereals, pasta, rice, new organic products, and vegetables. Most grown-up ladies ought to get around 21 grams of fiber daily.

Eat leafy foods. Have at any rate 1/2 cups of products of the soil cups of vegetables every day.

Understand names. Utilize the bundle mark data to help yourself settle on the most ideal decisions for a sound way of life.

Drink a lot of water. When in doubt, drink eight glasses of water each day. That satisfies the everyday necessity for most solid grown-ups.

Keep a solid weight. In case you're overweight, cut down on parcel estimates and eat fewer food varieties that are high in fat. Try not to skip dinners, however. An enrolled dietitian or your primary care physician can help you sort out your optimal body weight.

Scale back high-fat food sources. Fat ought to give 25% to 35% or less of your absolute everyday calories. Additionally, limit immersed fat to under 7% of your all-out day-by-day calories. Immersed fat raises cholesterol and lifts your danger for coronary illness. It's found in greasy meats, entire milk, frozen yogurt, and cheddar. Limit cholesterol to 300 milligrams or less each day. Furthermore, keep an eye out for trans fats, found in vegetable oils, many prepared merchandise, and some margarine. Trans fat likewise raises cholesterol and builds your danger for coronary illness.

Use sugar and salt with some restraint. An excessive amount of sodium in the eating regimen is connected to hypertension. Additionally, back off of smoked, salt-restored, and charbroiled food sources - these food sources have undeniable degrees of nitrates, which have been connected to the disease.

Limit liquor to one or fewer beverages daily

FOOD SOURCES TO HELP MENOPAUSE SIDE EFFECTS

Plant-based food varieties that have is flavones (plant estrogens) work in the body like a powerless type of estrogen. Consequently, soy may help soothe menopause manifestations, although exploration results are hazy. Some may help lower cholesterol levels and have been proposed to mitigate hot blazes and night sweats. Is flavones can be found in food sources, for example, tofu and soy milk.

Keep away from Food varieties During Menopause?

In case you're having hot blazes during menopause, you may discover it assists with staying away from certain "trigger" food sources and beverages, similar to fiery food varieties, caffeine, and liquor.

Enhancements After Menopause

Since there is an immediate connection between the absence of estrogen after menopause and the improvement of osteoporosis, the accompanying enhancements, joined with a solid eating regimen, may help forestall the beginning of this condition:

• Calcium If you think you need to take an enhancement to get sufficient calcium, check with your PCP first. A recent report recommends that taking calcium enhancements may raise the danger for cardiovascular failures in certain individuals - however, the investigation showed that expanding calcium in the eating routine through food sources didn't appear to raise the danger.

• Vitamin D. Your body utilizes nutrient D to assimilate calcium. Individuals ages 51 to 70 ought to get 600 IU every day. Those more than 70 ought to get 800 IU day by day. Over 4,000 IU of nutrient D, every day isn't suggested, because it might hurt the kidneys and debilitate bones.

SYNOPSIS FOUR

TAKING CHARGE OF THE CHANGE IN YOU

• Girls for the most part begin finding out about adolescence and the progressions coming up for them and their bodies in primary school, regularly years before the monthly cycle happens. Numerous eager moms begin investigating the intricate details of pregnancy and post-pregnancy issues before they at any point consider. Menopause, then again, appears to sneak up on numerous generally exhaustive and decidedly ready ladies, leaving them flushed, restless, touchy… and confounded.

• Dr. Stephanie , head of the Mayo Center's Office of Ladies' Wellbeing in Rochester and clinical proofreader of The Menopause Arrangement, sees numerous ladies who go to her griping of issues dozing, sporadic periods, or memory and fixation issues, stressed that there's something truly amiss with them. "Ladies are not anticipating this," says experts. "I have patients going to the Mayo Facility to sort out what's going on with them, and they're simply in per menopause [the quite a long while paving the way to menopause, during which chemical creation becomes unpredictable and less predictable]. They ask, 'For what reason didn't somebody advise me?'"

• As with adolescence and pregnancy, understanding what is befalling your body—and what can be done—diminishes the pressure of adapting to the going with changes. Like those other hormonal changes, encounters and indications of menopause fluctuate from one lady to another. A minority of menopausal ladies won't encounter recognizable or troublesome manifestations, while the greater part will encounter a mix of hot blazes, night sweats, weight acquire, weariness, rest unsettling influences, disposition changes, and changes in sexual capacity, to differing degrees.

These signs last only, around seven years, and now and then over 10 years. Ouch.

• The uplifting news is that we know more today than any other time about how to facilitate the indications of menopause. Menopause isn't an infection. Yet, on the off chance that a lady is encountering huge manifestations that ought not to be disregarded. We can treat those things. That is welcome information for the more than 2,000,000 ladies who enter menopause consistently, especially since expanding daily routine hopes imply that ladies are currently experiencing 33% of their lives past menopause. "The normal future for a lady in the mid-twentieth century was 50. This is an exciting modern lifestyle. Ladies didn't use to live for a very long time after menopause; we're actually attempting to sort out what that implies."

• Hormone substitution treatment has for quite some time been one of the go-to medicines for menopausal indications. The principal oral plan of estrogen was advertised in 1942, and from that point forward a great many menopausal ladies have utilized developing types of chemical treatment to treat their side effects. In any case, an extraordinary preventative banner was raised with the 2002 arrival of the Ladies' Wellbeing Drive (WHI) study results, which demonstrated that the utilization of the business chemical substitution treatment famous during the 1990s (explicitly, a medication called Preemptor, a blend of formed equine estrogen integrated from pregnant female horses' pee and engineered progestin) was connected with an expanded danger of coronary failure, stroke, blood clusters, and intrusive bosom malignancy. The discoveries sent stun waves through the clinical local area, and large numbers of the ones who had been utilizing chemical treatment deserted it.

• The study, which followed more than 160,000 postmenopausal ladies between the ages of 50–79, has since been the objective of analysis and reconsideration, as it has become certain that its outcomes in more established menopausal ladies were summed up—without logical premise—to more youthful menopausal ladies also. (The normal age for ladies in the investigation was 63—past the normal period of menopause beginning.) It likewise just tried a solitary financially accessible chemical mix that was well known at that point (Prempro), at a solitary, orally conveyed portion.

• "The WHI specialists were good-natured, yet the examination had some potentially negative results, we're actually attempting to compensate for that. An age of ladies botched the chance to take chemical treatment that required it, and we missed preparing an age of clinical professionals, who mastered something wrong." Today, most specialists concur that the advantages of chemical treatment exceed the dangers for ladies in their 50s who are inside 10 years of their last period and are encountering annoying side effects of menopause.

• Hormone treatment alternatives accessible today likewise work out in a good way past the oral engineered chemical definition included in the WHI study. Transdermal estrogen can be conveyed through skin creams or fixes (potentially alleviating certain dangers by bypassing the stomach-related parcel and the liver), and low-portion neighborhood vaginal estrogen treatment can be utilized to calm vaginal dryness. What's more, a few ladies like to utilize "bio identical" chemicals got from plants, which turned out to be all the more generally accessible in the mid-2000s in the wake of the WHI study and are indistinguishable in atomic construction to the chemicals normally delivered in a lady's body.

• "Understanding what is befalling your body decreases the pressure of changes."

• There's likewise ordinary fussing to facilitate the pressure and distress of menopause manifestations. Ringer drives a six-week "shared clinical visit" at the Penny George Foundation for gatherings of up to 10 menopausal ladies, offering them the opportunity to interface and get support from ladies encountering comparable manifestations, just as find out about comprehensive ways to deal with treatment, including spices and enhancements, reflection, sustenance, Chinese medication, and fragrant healing. "It will in general be very certifying for the ones who take an interest," says Ringer. "Notwithstanding their shifted foundations, there's a connectedness and appreciation that improves their capacity to deal with their menopause."

• While some researchers advocates for the advantages of chemical treatment to moderate manifestations of menopause, she additionally sees a lot of ladies who have sufficient achievement utilizing elective, non-drug strategies that they don't have to think about it. Restricting the utilization of prepared food varieties, desserts, caffeine, and liquor, for example, can diminish the seriousness of hot glimmers in certain ladies, as can pressure decrease strategies, exercise, and spices like dark cohosh (an individual from the buttercup family).

• Researchers stress that, while menopausal indications can be a test, the change into post-menopause can be a freeing and cheerful season of life. "Numerous individuals in our way of life approach maturing with fear," says Ringer. "Yet, I like to discuss the part of astuteness and advantages of involvement that accompanies it. Similarly, there's a stupendous shift that occurs with adolescence and pregnancy, menopause can be a positive change in life that accompanies a feeling of shrewdness and another stage."

• "It's a period you can venture back and reevaluate and rethink, Think about every one of the ones who got popular after 50—Julia Youngster, Mother Teresa, Georgia O'Keeffe. On the off chance that you need to go take a craftsmanship class, in case you're miserable in your work, if there's something you've for a long while been itching to do, presently the time. The standards have changed; it's a significant achievement and an opportunity to pursue the existence you truly need."

CONCLUTION

In the event that you're a woman, you in all probability understand that our bodies go through bundle changes over the span of our lives. Synthetic compounds expect an irreplaceable part in those movements at each period of progress, from pubescence to post-menopause.

After entering the world, levels of these synthetic compounds are high, yet they decrease a few months and stay low until puberty]. During pre-adulthood, real changes in the body are overseen by changes in the levels of synthetic substances that are being made. In early puberty, compound levels augment and strengthen the making of sex synthetics (the synthetic compounds in the body that control pubescence and multiplication), including estrogen. This extension in estrogen causes real changes related to immaturity in youngsters, including improvement of the chests, ovaries, uterus, and vagina, similarly as a young woman's first period.

The ordinary time of pubescence starting in youngsters is 10-and-a-half years old, yet it can go from seven to 13 years old, with menarche (a young woman's first ladylike cycle) occurring at around 12-and-a-half to 13 years of age. African-American and

Hispanic youngsters will overall start youth imperceptibly sooner than Caucasian young women. The entire pattern of pubescence in youngsters takes approximately three to four years.

Month to month time periods continues until per menopause, the stage in life which is ordinarily depicted as when a women's body begins changing to menopause. Per menopause, which can continue to go for a long time, conventionally begins when a woman is in her late forties, anyway it can start earlier or later. During per menopause, the period ends up being less typical and a woman can experience night sweats, bother resting, hot flickers, vaginal dryness, and outlook issues.

Menopause is, clearly, an ordinary piece of development that every woman will go through, generally by her mid-fifties. The synthetic substances estrogen and progesterone, which control the month-to-month cycle, will decrease during this time, achieving less conventional periods. Likewise, a woman's ovaries will stop conveying eggs into the fallopian tubes.

Lightning Source UK Ltd.
Milton Keynes UK
UKHW020958100821
388622UK00015B/1202

9 798517 437242